SELF HEALING DYNAMICS

FOR CANCER AND OTHER ILLNESSES

JAN KING GARVERICK

MORGANA PUBLICATIONS
P.O. BOX 5403
EVANSTON, ILLINOIS 60204 - 5403

Copyright © 1992 by Jan Garverick

All rights reserved. No part of this book may be reproduced or transmitted in any form or by any means, electronic or mechanical, including photocopying, recording or by any informational storage or retrieval system—except by a reviewer who may quote brief passages in a review to be printed in a magazine or newspaper—without permission in writing from the publisher. For information contact **Morgana Publications,** P.O. Box 5403, Evanston, Illinois 60204 - 5403.

First printing 1992

Although the author and publisher have exhaustively researched all sources to ensure the accuracy and completeness of the information contained in this book, we assume no responsibility for errors, inaccuracies, omissions, or any inconsistency herein. Any slights of people or organizations are unintentional. Readers should use their own judgment or consult a holistic medical expert or their personal physicians for specific applications to their individual problems.

ISBN 0-9630177-0-5

Editor: June Rouse
Cover Design: Elaine Morales
Typesetting: Sandstone Graphics
Morton Grove

CONTENTS

Acknowledgments v

Poem vii

Introduction 1

Chapter 1
Come Along With Me 5
    An invitation to discover new ways to use our creativity to enhance our health

Chapter 2
Doctors............................... 13
    Coming to terms with love/hate relationships based on childhood experiences

Chapter 3
Hodgkins 17
    Combining traditional medical practices and augmentive approaches to wellness bring successful results

Chapter 4
Visualization and Other Miracles 21
    A new way to use early childhood fantasies

Chapter 5
Massage: The Magic of Touch............. 25
    Another spoke in the wheel of wellness

Chapter 6
What is This Thing Called "Exercise"?....... 29
    Love of sports becomes a valuable asset to regain strength

Chapter 7
Nutrition: Learning to Care 35
    Eating for fun adds new dimension to old habits

Chapter 8
Humor, A Big Surprise 41
    Laughter: A daily Rx for radiant health

Chapter 9
Tears and Rage 45
    Emotions and the necessity to release them

Chapter 10
Energy: Not Seeing is Believing 49
    Using energy concepts in the healing process

Chapter 11
Meditation 55
    Bringing the busy mind to a state of peacefulness

Chapter 12
Journaling 59
    A regular discipline that's rewarding and fun

Chapter 13
Inner dialoguing.......................... 63
    Listening to your heart

Chapter 14
Life's Purpose and Passion 69
    Living life fully, savoring each moment

Chapter 15
The Doctor of the Future 75
    Guess who?

Chapter 16
Commitment 81
    Begin it now!

Selected Bibliography 86

ACKNOWLEDGMENTS

Thanks from my heart to all who believed in me, all my "healthy nags" who insisted I complete this book. I especially want to honor each and every person who left this life as a result of cancer or cancer-related illnesses; for they are my true inspiration to share my own story, my struggles for aliveness, my decisions to participate in my prognosis, and my joyous movement **from illness to wellness**.

Special thanks to Mary Gynn and Barbara Osborne, my soul sisters, to daughters Nicole and Trina Goetz, who are my shining lights, their father Greg, and to Don Tuskey, my earth mate and soul mate. Thanks also to my loved ones near and far who constantly stood by me when I doubted myself, especially June Rouse, Carol Owens, Harriet Porter, Bob McClellan and Anne Cleary. And I will always remember the beacons of light in the medical arena, Drs. Maylahn, Messmore and Knaus.

This book is dedicated to my mother,
Helen King Chalupka, my dear teacher, and my father, Stanley
Chalupka and his wife Ellen, who teach me about love.
Most of all, it's dedicated to the
connection we all have to our one
source of truth, the Inner Voice.

CANVAS OF LIFE

A fresh new piece of canvas
starts the tender life newborn,
and every moment lived thereon,
new colors will adorn.

Royal purple—our first step.
Our first heartache—midnight blue.
A bold stroke here, a speckle there,
our every dream another hue.

All our lives creating,
with every smile and every tear,
with every lesson, good and bad,
new, graceful strokes appear.

And you and I creators
who paint this work of art.
Choosing every step with care
to best portray our heart.

Believe you only hold the brush
that paints your canvas bright,
and before you lies your future
on a canvas, clean and white.

—Trina Goetz

INTRODUCTION

Much time has passed since I was first diagnosed with Hodgkins, a form of cancer classified as a "lymphoma." Fifteen years later, I have a radically different perspective on my personal experience with a major, life-threatening illness; I now understand that the process of recovery is not always "speedy" as the greeting card companies would have us believe. For one thing, recovery, or *survival* as I have come to call it, means different things to different people. For me, survival means thinking of myself as less of a victim and more of a winner. It means actively making decisions regarding my health and wellness, not passively allowing others, including well-meaning relatives and doctors, to dictate my treatment.

"Victims," as I see it, feel helpless, even hopeless. This manual offers a variety of options and choices so that we (including those currently afflicted with cancer and other illnesses) can feel that we are participating in, and even directing, the outcome of our illnesses and of our lives.

We will speak of *healing*, which, again, is defined by each of us in vastly different ways. One person's healing may be a peaceful acceptance of death; another's healing may be working with those who are similarly afflicted. Healing, therefore, does not necessarily mean being disease-free, although it certainly could mean that. You alone will uncover what healing uniquely means to you. Consider this manual a menu, one from which you can select options and ideas to construct your own unparalleled healing.

1
COME ALONG WITH ME

This isn't a book about cancer. It is about how I survived it and how I now live with the freedom and assurance that my experience with cancer is a valuable, yet distinct part of my past. Yes, it was an ordeal, a very real one, fifteen years ago when I was diagnosed as having Hodgkins at the age of thirty-five; but enough time has passed so that while I remember most of the details, the actual event seems to have happened to another person. During the three years after my diagnosis, I survived an exploratory surgery, a spleenectomy (spleem removal), a month of radiation therapy, a laparotomy (removal of a lobe of the lung) and chemotherapy (in that order). Interspersed were varieties of x-rays, diagnostic tests, EKG's, and countless other probings. By the time my last treatment, the chemotherapy, ended over twelve years ago, I was beginning to feel disease-free, although the doctors never called me *cured*.

Although my body showed no further signs of disease, I was filled with doubts and fears that have taken years to overcome. It took me another twelve years to *feel* cured mentally and emotionally. Preparing to die was one matter; learning to live, quite another! A stranger began to emerge in the mirror, and I didn't really know her.

In many ways, you see, I actually *became* another person. I did this through exciting, often demanding inner work. By inner work, I mean seeking to strengthen my inner core of beliefs about myself and others; simply put, by learning to love myself enough to use discipline and choice to stay happy and healthy. All along the way, this has meant not letting others make decisions for me and not letting myself be miserable because of what someone else is doing, or not doing. And acquiring and developing the following disciplines, though not as simple as they may sound, certainly helped make my recovery possible:

Visualization Integrative body work
Meditation   Dream interpretation
Massage   Journaling

I also reintroduced myself to something I hadn't done since junior high school, something called physical exercise (done faithfully). My life also includes "intuitive nutrition," or being finely tuned to the body's nutritional needs, letting the body itself determine exactly what to eat and not to eat. The final ingredient to my magic formula for radiant health is laughter—and plenty of it!

How Did I Get Sick?

Since early childhood, perhaps going back as far as life in the womb, certain thought patterns develop. Through the years, anger, resentment, guilt and grief and all the conditions related to these feelings build up or accumulate. A great deal of research has shown that these low energy thought patterns cause stress, depress the immune system and can eventually cause illness. I believe my own low energy conditions were very damaging and, in fact, nearly killed me. I wasn't going to let myself die at the age of thirty-five—not if I could help it! I began to realize that I *could* help—I could help myself by changing the way I looked at life. A very serious commitment to this change would be required in order to get to the bottom of the "baggage" I had collected since birth.

According to Wayne Dyer and Brough Joy, cancer patients tend to withdraw into themselves, feeling closed off from others and very alone. I wanted to understand how I chose the punishment of illness by focusing on emotions that fostered a sense of aloneness and abandonment. Bit by bit, slowly, painfully, and resisting my own better judgment every step of the way, I have learned what health and freedom are. I have created a cancer-free lifestyle, and now I want to share this formula of freedom with others.

Will You Accept the Challenge?

To those who now have or have had cancer: It is my heartfelt wish that you will read this book and glean from it whatever disciplines and practices will add dimension to your current lifestyle. Experiment with them and customize them to your own uniqueness.

Create your own formula for a healthy, joyful life by relying on your creativity and intuitiveness. Choose your perfect system for living. Most of all, be patient with your progress...for the belief systems which create cancer are often insidious and deeply engrained in the subconscious mind. The subconscious mind is that part of the mind that stores all your experiences and, often ruled by fear and lovelessness, chatters endlessly about everything you **should** and **shouldn't** do and be. Replacing that loveless chatter with positive, peaceful thoughts requires dedication and commitment to all you believe you can be. It can be done, say Dr. Bernie Siegel and actor-comedian Joe Kogel, who go around the world teaching that the human spirit can overcome anything.

Many miracles occur in the healing process. These miracles require but one ingredient: A WILLINGNESS TO HEAL. To those of you who feel hopeless or helpless, I urge you to continue to explore the options and exercises in the following chapters. Agree to turn one page after another and read this book. Who knows, you may stumble upon a miracle.

Fear of Someday

For those of you who have never had cancer, yet live in the fear that someday it will strike: This book is required reading. Somehow, up to now, you have managed to compensate for the fear of getting cancer. You have eluded "it," dodged "it" or otherwise outsmarted "it." In your mind cancer is a mysterious beast that may someday grab hold of you. It's a bogeyman that's hiding in the closet, waiting to pounce on you when you're distracted. You live life with tension and fear, knowing that if you let down your guard, your shell, for even one second, you'll be devoured.

You are the people with lots of promise. You have grit, determination and cunning; you know how to survive and, while your survival formula has a few glitches in it, it's gotten you this far. You have the foundation for a long and healthy life. You are the fortunate ones, who can teach others by your example. The relatively healthy body you inhabit may have an ulcer or two, allergies every spring, asthma, herpes, tooth decay, and an assortment of other diseases and maladies, but you have avoided the killer diseases. I salute you. But read on; there's much to learn. Your life can be restructured in such a way that cancer will no longer be a threat to you. All the grit and energy you use to fight the so-called "dragon" can be channeled into what you've always wanted: A LIFE OF FREEDOM AND JOY.

An Invitation

To those of you who have never had cancer and know you never will: I invite you to come out of the closet and show others your lifestyle. Teach us your secrets for living exquisitely. You know who you are. You are in health clubs teaching fitness, counselors for abused children, in the pathology labs studying disease. You are artists and poets with messages of light and love. You are surgeons sweating over yet another life, working fourteen hour days. You are the Mexican gardeners and the Illinois soybean farmers, the gas station attendants, the massage therapists who lovingly touch AIDS patients. You are the psychologists and therapists who counsel incest survivors and substance abusers. You are the famous and infamous politicians and leaders, the union and non-union schoolteachers and steelworkers. You are businessmen in pin-striped suits, stockbrokers in the pit and lawyers in hearings.

You are every man and any woman who has chosen in your silent or not-so-silent ways to teach others. You are open to learn from them, as well, that life is to be lived with zest; and that once you have learned to serve yourselves, serving others is the key to fulfillment.

Join with me in your unique ways. Tell us how you live life with zeal. What makes you happy and alive? What makes energy course through your body so that five or six hours of sleep a night is enough? How do you create? I invite you to read my formula for a cancer-free life. Edit it. Amend it. Write your own books. Or live your life with that silent, serene eloquence that needs no words. You won't lose your identity by looking at healing with new eyes; you will have gained it, brought it into the light for others to see. You will have shared yourself. You will have become my partner in the journey!

2
DOCTORS

Since birth, I have had a love/hate relationship with doctors. I was a home delivery baby, which meant no anesthetic for my mom. It also meant my grandmother was an assistant at the event. The doctor who delivered me also became my pediatrician. When I became three, Dr. Carter seemed stern and serious. He never cracked even the hint of a smile. Even at the age of three, I considered **every** part of my anatomy "necessary," and he was the culprit who relieved me of a very necessary part of my anatomy, my tonsils! Surgical removal of *anything* constituted a violation that holds to this day. I was outraged that Dr. Carter and my mother made decisions without consulting me. I felt helpless.

Some years later I was awakened in what seemed like the middle of the night by my mother and our "new" family doctor. He happened to be my mother's cousin, but his appearance at my bedside was terrorizing. Mom and the doctor were examining what turned out to be a hernia, although mom thought it was a tumor. It, too, had to be removed, they decided. Once again, I fell victim to radical decisions about my precious body that were made by my caretakers and not by me. It could very well be that, at the tender age of five, I developed a deep fear of tumors within my subconscious mind—a fear that would surface thirty years later.

Up to this point, my short history with doctors did not endear them to me. Every time one came near me, a portion of my anatomy was removed, and with great physical pain. I felt violated and assaulted by doctors. A feeling of helplessness arose every time I looked at a stethoscope and a white jacket, a feeling that was to continue throughout my adult life.

Minor surgeries and two babies later, at the age of thirty, every time I walked into a doctor's office I gave myself to him, body and soul. I never participated in decisions regarding my body. The doctor was *God,* at least God of my physical world. It never occurred to me to disagree with doctors or even to discuss options for treatment. In fact, when my children were little, I became so engrossed in their well being that I neglected, even denied, my own health. I smoked and drank excessively, thinking no one noticed; any bodily pain or discomfort were deferred to "motherhood," and certainly not discussed with anyone, especially my husband who seemed more and more distracted with his work. Depression set in, and, one month before my thirty-fifth birthday I knew something was very, very wrong with me!

3
HODGKINS

At the age of thirty-five, my world collapsed. After many months of knowing something was "wrong", I was diagnosed with Hodgkins, a form of cancer that can be deadly. My two daughters were six and eight years old. My marriage was headed for the rocks. Not a good time!

I would have a chance to get to know doctors of all kinds—at close range. Mayo Clinic in Rochester, Minnesota, was the place I chose for my first surgery. There, a saint of a man decided to operate on my chest tumor based on, of all things, *aesthetics*. He didn't want a thirty-five year old woman to have an ugly scar, so he opted for an incision that curved along the rib cage and under the arm instead of a frontal incision through my sternum. The surgery turned out to be exploratory; with his sensitive decision to perform the less radical surgical procedure, that doctor possibly saved my life. The tumor was inoperable and radiation therapy was required. To this day I believe that, considering my condition at that time, a radical frontal incision would have meant my life.

Slowly, I began to realize that people called doctors, whom I had learned to fear and hate as a child, included men and women who cared about more than the purely physical aspects of their patients' well being. I learned to say "yes" or "no" to the various treatments that were offered. I had choices. The more educated I became about the world of medicine and the form and function of my own body, the more capable I was to participate in and to prescribe my own cure. Having let others determine my destiny for thirty-five years, I needed time to experiment with this new concept of self-responsibility. The reality of having cancer was such a frightening motivator that I opted for all the help I could get, and that included my feelings about doctors. I found myself taking them down from their godlike pedestals and placing them in positions of advisors and allies. They became loving guides who would assist me back to wholeness and health.

And, I began to ask questions, lots of questions, of anyone in a white jacket. I wanted to know everything about my illness, all the details, all the statistics. I absorbed every bit of it; my brain whirled with input. I welcomed each new white jacket as the bearer of precious data to put into my research hopper. Somewhere in the midst of everything, my inner self made a decision to do WHATEVER WAS NECESSARY TO BE HEALTHY AND WHOLE AGAIN. That included serious consideration of all the medical facts and figures. In my current physical condition, I knew I had to do more than *wish* myself back to health. I needed doctors, nurses, all the technology to measure my progress. And, I needed surgery and medication even though the thought of either revolted me.

For the first time in my life I saw doctors working with me instead of against me. We became friends; we became one. Our mission was total health for me. I had several reasons to stay alive and get healthy. My marriage needed a decision and my children needed raising. Pain lay ahead, but beyond it stood the promise of recovery and survival. I knew with all my heart that pleasure would follow. But first, the pain. I had to step through it. Just about then, someone handed me a book on, of all things, *visualization.*

4
VISUALIZATION and OTHER MIRACLES

As a young child, I had a very active imagination. I would sit on the porch in the afternoon sun with my paper dolls, dressing them and taking them places in my mind. I created lengthy conversations about the spice of life. My paper dolls were very real to me. No distinction existed for me between what is termed real and unreal. My imagination was a part of me that I never questioned, at least not at the age of five.

Yet now, at the age of thirty-five, as I started to read more and more books about imagery and visualization, I was skeptical. Sure, the books described how people were getting amazing results with cancer using these techniques, but I couldn't make the connection about how a mental picture could affect the body in any way. Could drawing a picture of my tumor eliminate it, or reduce it? That didn't make sense. I had forgotten how real the world of my imagination once had been. I was an adult woman with a very big challenge and I was scared! Maybe I was scared enough to try anything.

By the time I had chemotherapy, I had a new husband and a new home in Ohio. My mother-in-law showed me a book by Leslie and O. Carl Simonton called *Getting Well Again*. It has become the standard bearer for imagery work with cancer patients. At this time, the premise of patients participating in their own cure through visualization was relatively new and unproven. Yet I knew visualization would work for me. Along with the chemotherapy, I visualized pink and blue cancer cells being spread on a toast-like slab, cut into quarters and scraped out of my body forever. This is the way I saw it, and I imaged this scene again and again. I even found a little piece of carpet padding that looked just like my image. I snipped it off to carry in my purse as a reminder to do my visualization exercise.

To this day I don't know how it worked. Which was it, the chemotherapy or my mental imagery that freed my body of cancer? Was it a little of both? Miracles can't be proven, but I now have perfect health and that can be proven. How I got that way is still a mystery, yet I know somehow that visualization played a part.

■■■■■■■■■■■■■■■■■■■■■■■■■■■■■■■

VISUALIZATION EXERCISE

The following exercise is the first of a series that follow each chapter. You will find them to be very helpful in understanding and experiencing the chapter's focus. This exercise is best done when you have a half hour or more to yourself.

1. Fill your bathtub with comfortably warm water.

2. If you wish, you may light candles and/or play soft music.

3. Enjoy your bath for as long as you wish.
4. When you are ready to get out of the tub, remain there and pull the plug.
5. Sit in the tub as the water runs out, visualizing that all your anger, pain and/or illness, anything unpleasant that you want to get rid of, are running out of the tub with the water.
6. Continue to see your _____ (you fill in whatever you have chosen to visualize being washed down the drain) until the water has completely run out of the tub.
7. Let yourself be in touch with how your body feels sitting in the empty tub.
8. Repeat this exercise whenever you feel a need to release anything that is unpleasant, such as anger, pain and even a specific illness—anything that you wish to no longer have. Just say as the water drains out of the tub, "I see my _____ going down the drain. The water is carrying my anger down the drain and away from me. I relax in comfort and I feeel good."

NOTE: This exercise may be done using a shower, also.

5
MASSAGE: THE MAGIC of TOUCH

Another miracle that came into my life as I lay recuperating in Ohio that summer was a gift from my young daughters, Nicole and Trina. In a town of 500 inhabitants, including cats and dogs, the only place to go for excitement was the library twenty miles away. One excursion turned up a book on massage. Nicole and Trina wanted to learn massage. Since I spent much of my day in bed, they had a captive audience and a most grateful recipient. I was the guinea pig. Trina would work on my hands and Nicole would take a foot. We laughed a lot. I felt good being massaged and waited excitedly for them to return from school to practice on me.

I became a junkie to feeling good and gradually learned that I needed less and less of my pain prescriptions. Life became very precious, and I didn't want to miss any of it. Slowly, very slowly, the pain which was part of my daily existence diminished. Massage seemed to be a pain reliever in and of itself!

To this day, I consider it a miracle that my daughters and I discovered the healing process of massage. None of us ever had experienced massage, nor were there any massage therapists in the family. What is more, neither my ex-husband nor I came from a family of "touchers". In fact, our backgrounds were more those of non-expressive families. Yet in that warm Ohio summer, my daughters and I discovered a miracle of touch that has been a part of our lives ever since.

■■■■■■■■■■■■■■■■■■■■■■■■■■■■■■■■■■

MASSAGE EXERCISES

1. Call your local massage association (American Massage Therapy Association is one) and get the name of a qualified massage therapist in your area. Have a professional massage regularly!

2. Ask a buddy to exchange back or foot massages with you. You don't have to be an "expert" to enjoy the magic of touch. Do this often!

3. The next time you are with a group of friends, make a "massage train" by sitting in a row behind each other so that each person massages the back of the person sitting in front of him/her. This is also lots of fun in a big circle.

4 You might even consider taking a massage class at a local learning center. It's fun and, who knows, you may decide to embark on a new career!

6
WHAT IS THIS THING CALLED "EXERCISE"?

As a child, I was always physically active. I rode a bicycle as soon as I could walk, climbed trees and ran early in life. I even played baseball and football. Back in the fifties, girls who played baseball or football were called "tomboys." In the eighties they were called Olympic contenders. Things changed. But in my early years, exercise generally was not equated with good health. So as I became a "woman" I gave up sports for more "feminine" attributes such as cooking. The feminist movement had not emerged. I acquiesced to the dictates of my time.

Throughout both marriages I lurked around the fringes of athletics. In Illinois the public swimming pool was two miles away. I bicycled there daily, even taking my first child on a baby carrier through the eighth month of my second pregnancy. I was physically fit in those days. But after that, the needs of my children came first. They had swimming lessons at the local YMCA, and I neglected myself. Being a mother meant sacrificing my own needs, or so I thought.

Many years later, right in the middle of chemotherapy, I rediscovered swimming and tennis. My new husband, Trent, would take me to the tennis courts saying, "Come on, sissy. Lob the ball as if you mean it!" My stomach wrenched with pain whenever I reached out to stroke the ball. "I'll show him I'm no sissy," I thought, ever the tough competitor. Every minute was pain. Parts of my lungs had forgotten what air felt like. They rebelled. The chemotherapy sessions made me nauseous and limp and exerting activities like tennis challenged every cell of my being.

Trent continued to taunt me. He was relentless, even cruel and heartless, I thought. Today I see him as an angel sent to inspire me with hope; hope that my body would be strong again, just as it was when I played football in the backyards of my New England childhood.

Progress was slow. I became discouraged. The pain of my illness and the pain of my recovery merged into a mass of confusion. I didn't know what to believe about my body. Was I recovering or was I dying? Were doctors and loved ones telling me the truth? What was the truth? Did anyone know? Did I know? And if I didn't, then who did?

In the middle of great doubt and fear, the survivor instinct emerged. With the first sign of snow, I began to think of skiing Before Hodgkins, I was a strong intermediate alpine skier. Could I do it again? The thought frightened me. Skiing was demanding. It required great stamina and skill. Would my body remember the precise stops and turns?

My doctor encouraged me. He was amused by my daring prescriptions for wellness. When I had asked him about weightlifting the previous year, he laughed, "Go ahead and try it. You're a spunky woman. You seem to know what's best for you."

That winter I skied every slope in Michigan. The next spring

31

I skied Utah, the following year, Colorado. It was glorious to stand on a black diamond slope atop Mt. Ajax in Aspen, knowing I had completed the run and would do it again.

I became self-directed, knowing only I could create my reality and my recovery. Those mountains birthed a spiritual quest that has never stopped. I found a special force in those mountain pines, and a power within myself. Was this what people called freedom?

Since then I have taken up running and swimming, taught fitness in a health club and became a certified boardsailor. My new activities require no prescription, and I custom mix and match them to suit the seasons. Moreover, the feeling of pride for having learned a new skill lets me know that I'm in charge of my life. Instead of checking everything out with my doctors, I have become aware of what my body can handle. Its powers and capabilities are simply amazing!

■ ■

EXERCISE EXERCISES

1. Start small. Choose an exercise that is "do-able." Be realistic. Consider your physical condition. Walking for ten or fifteen minutes two times a week is a good start. Set the same time each day to take your walk. The main point is to be consistent. Set a realistic goal and stick to it. If you are in good physical condition and are not recovering from surgery, choose more challenging goals such as jogging, aerobics or swimming three or four times a week.

2. Monitor your body, what it can and cannot do. You will begin to learn how far you can push it safely. There may be discomfort and resistance, but once you begin to see changes and improvements in your stamina and endurance, you will be greatly encouraged to go for more.

3 Set new goals as you progress. Allow for backsliding. It's only human. Keep on keeping on. You'll love yourself for it. Most of all, have fun with yourself as you become good friends with your body.

7
NUTRITION: LEARNING TO CARE

As a child, I was a finicky eater. To me meat was "yucky," but with two parents of eastern European heritage, meats and sausages were daily fare. They were our soul food, so to speak. Everyone thought meats were essential elements of nutrition back in the '40s and '50s. American health standards promoted the basic four food groups and protein was king.

At the age of ten, I discovered that living things had to be slaughtered in order to put meat on the table. My revulsion for meat made sense. It was inhumane to me. I refused to eat meat. My mother gave me protein supplements so I wouldn't die. I still refused to eat meat.

Like other principles in my life, my vegetarian beliefs got lost in the need for acceptance and love. My husband insisted on meat every day and I dutifully prepared and ate it. My passions and principles were lost in the energy I spent being what others wanted me to be. More and more I wanted to please others, less and less myself. Who was I, really? Arguing about food seemed so petty. I just wanted to be loved. I'd have eaten grilled boa constrictor if that meant someone would love me!

The subject of food never came up for me again until I was getting radiation therapy. My appetite left completely. That's when my inner voice, as I call it, kicked in. I started to ask my thinning body what to eat, and I started to listen. "Cottage cheese." "Mixed vegetables." "Broccoli." These were the foods my body wanted. I'd hear this little voice in my head and sure enough, cottage cheese tasted great. So did vegetables, especially broccoli, along with fruits and sprouts. My family objected to my new eating habits. Surely I would lose more weight if I continued with this silly "listen to my body" diet.

But I was in a survival mode and overrode my family's objections. I followed my inner voice and slowly began to regain the weight I had lost. Little did my family know that less than ten years later, Professor T. C. Campbell, senior science advisor to the American Institute for Cancer Research would acknowledge "a strong correlation between dietary protein intake and cancer of the breast, prostate, pancreas, and colon." And a year after that, Myron Winick, Director of Columbia University's Institute of Human Nutrition, would say that data indicates "a relationship between high-protein diets and cancer of the colon."

I now have become a vegan, one who eats vegetable foods only, including such things as tofu, tempeh and miso, words I couldn't even pronounce back then. Dairy products and sugar are no longer part of my diet, but I have learned 57 ways to fix tofu.

Being a vegetarian gives me more energy. I had always been an eight-hour-a-night sleeper. Now, six hours of sleep is maximum. But moving from a meat eater to veganism wasn't an overnight process.

In the 1980s I was in the heat of a corporate sales position and focused very little on food. Yet I began to decline the prime rib dinners in favor of fish. Slowly my awareness of nutrition evolved; my body responded with more aliveness than I'd ever known.

Many excellent nutrition books will assist you in fine tuning your eating experience. *Fit For Life* by Marilyn and Harvey Diamond and *Eat to Win* by Dr. Robert Haas are two. Dr. Haas is a clinical nutritionist who counseled gymnast Martina Navritilova. One that will amaze you is John Robbins' *Diet For A New America*, which approaches vegetarianism from all angles, including animal rights and ecology.

Talk to your doctors and nurses, also, when gathering nutrition information, although doctors will be the first to admit they have very little knowledge of nutrition. More and more medical professionals are coming to realize, however, the importance of nutrition and are beginning to prescribe vitamins, minerals and other supplements as well.

Once again, be patient with yourself as you gather information. Your body may resent any radical dietary changes after all those years of indulgence! It will cry "Meat!" in the middle of the night (and it won't be your inner voice!). You may get the urge to drive to Haagen Dazs at midnight for a double scoop of pralines and cream. Love yourself for those cravings; it's only natural. The body has a memory like an elephant; it doesn't give up easily. Recently, I dreamed I was eating a thick juicy hamburger with raw onions. After eight years of vegetarianism, I still drool at the thought!

I have been known to consider homicide if someone ate my chocolate eclair. For me, caffeine and sugar are the last of the nasties to go (and they are nasties, robbing the body of nutrients). But you'll soon love the taste of "decaf", and even herbal teas will tempt you. Until last year, I was known to prowl the local 7-Eleven for a cup of half real coffee/half decaf at dubious hours of the day and night. If the craving hits you, humor yourself now and then. The time will come when saying "no" will be a more loving choice than saying "yes."

Eventually, discipline and commitment are required to maintain a healthy nutrition formula, but you'll like the way you feel after you've decided to focus on good eating practices. Customize the quality of your life by using nutrition to unlock the door to a cancer-free life. It's a critical key!

■ ■

NUTRITION EXERCISES

The following exercises are designed for FUN! You get to participate in gathering more information about a different way of eating, leaning toward vegetarianism. Be patient with yourself. Don't expect to make changes overnight (although some have). Changes in behavior, especially something as basic as eating, do take time. You may take two steps forward and one step back, but just stick with it! Try one or more of the following:

1. Visit a natural food store. Allow yourself plenty of time (at least an hour) to check it out. Pick things up, read labels, perhaps even purchase something new and interesting, something you've never eaten before.

2. Buy a vegetarian cookbook and cook a meal from it. (Give your family fair warning if you don't want a revolution on your hands!)

3. Take a vegetarian cooking class. It's becoming more popular than ever. Check your local community centers or local health and wellness magazines. Bon Appetit!

4. Visit a local vegetarian restaurant with a friend, preferably one that has been recommended to you by a seasoned vegetarian. All vegetarian restaurants aren't necessarily great, so it's a good idea to patronize a reputable establishment for your maiden voyage.

8
HUMOR, A BIG SURPRISE

In 1979, Norman Cousins wrote *Anatomy of an Illness*. In it, he reveals how laughter and humor affected his recovery from a crippling illness. Since then, much has been written about the role of humor and laughter in wellness.

A friend of mine who is a Registered Nurse and professional clown explains that in the state of laughter the body releases chemicals called tryptophan and endorphines. Besides making us feel good, these chemicals have a physiological effect on the heart and circulatory systems.

Discovering one has cancer is no laughing matter, but bringing laughter into one's life has proven results for even the most critically ill. Remember, the subconscious mind absorbs information like a sponge. Why not make that information positive and funny? *Fake* laughing if you have to! (And notice how you feel afterwards. If you just feel embarrassed, keep on laughing; the action of your laugh-muscles will set those good chemicals into action if you give it a chance.) Rent funny videos. Tell jokes. Ask people to tell you jokes instead of commenting about, or even **thinking about** how bad you look. Be outrageous. You have nothing to lose except your illness. (We still believe in miracles, remember?) Who knows, you may "live" laughing.

Cancer patients are known to take themselves very seriously. In fact, they generally take life seriously. You may have to teach yourself to laugh, and the best teacher is repetition. Keep doing it!

■■■■■■■■■■■■■■■■■■■■■■■■■■■■■■■■■■■

HUMOR EXERCISES

1. This exercise works best with three or more people. Lying on the floor have one person lie at a right angle to your head, then place your head on his/her stomach. Another person lies at right angle to your body and places his/her head on your stomach. Continue the chain for as many people as are in the group. Before you know it, someone in the group will have an irresistible urge to laugh, and the laughing chain reaction will be contageous.

2. Ever wonder which funny movies to rent? Here's a list of flicks guaranteed to leave you limp (and lighter) from laughter:
   Scrooged, Bill Murray
   Planes, Trains and Automobiles
   The Gods Must Be Crazy I and II
   Anything with Steve Martin
   Anything with Peter Sellers
   Anything with Chevy Chase

3. If you are physically fit and live near a metropolitan area, visit a local comedy house. Improvisational comedy is best, since there's always the element of surprise.

43

9
TEARS AND RAGE

Actually, crying is closely related to anger. When someone lets us down, we get angry. When we let ourselves down, we get angry at ourselves. And when the anger is expressed and released, in whatever way that is done, sadness is felt. If the sadness is allowed to be expressed, we cry.

Crying is the body's way of healing the hurt. Most of us are born crying. Who wouldn't cry after being forced out of the comfort and safety of a mother's womb? The original rejection! And once we begin to cry, we discover that crying actually feels good. We feel relieved. The buildup of chemicals that are the result of negative passions is released. Notice how babies both yell and cry at the same time. That's anger and sadness being expressed in its most natural state. Babies aren't embarrassed and they don't feel guilty about expressing themselves, either.

As we get older, the expression of emotion is less accepted. In fact, it's frowned upon. Now without getting into a lot of complicated psychological theory about exactly what emotions are and how they relate to self-actualization, I'm going to suggest that you incorporate the expression of anger and sadness into your everyday life. Beat pillows, shred newspaper, scream in the privacy of your home, get rip roaring mad. You might want to warn your family that this is coming. Also, tell them you're expressing a "nameless" anger which has nothing to do with them. It may, but trust me, now isn't the time to expend energy figuring out who did what to whom and was it in 1969. This is your life and, if you have anger, it's yours. What you need to do is get rid of it, safely for yourself and certainly safely for others. Talk to a counselor about how best to express and release emotion. In fact, I recommend counseling for the recovering cancer patient since issues of self-esteem often arise.

Moreover, don't deny the feelings, or push them down. Holding on to angry feelings creates a feeling of separation, and feeling separate actually creates illness.

The process of grieving, as expressed by human tears, is the most beautiful experience of all. Some say that tears wash the soul clean. Along with the tears comes forgiveness—of others, and, finally, of ourselves. As we allow ourselves to grieve and cry about our losses, we begin to feel lighter, at peace with ourselves, at peace with others. Feelings of oneness replace those of separation; cells actually heal in the body through grieving and tears. We become renewed and regenerated . We come to terms with ourselves. We let go.

■ ■

FEELINGS EXERCISES

I heartily recommend a good counselor or therapist to guide you as you begin to look at your feelings. Most of us expend a great deal of effort hiding our feelings. Uncovering them or letting them out is a very delicate matter. Seek professional support as you delve into the wonderful world of feelings. It is said that tears are the soul's way of washing itself; as you allow yourself to cry, you will feel lighter and freer.

Anger is a different matter. Most cancer patients have internalized their anger. You will definitely need guidance as you learn to redirect your anger AWAY from your own body. Learning to express anger is a tricky business, especially if you came from a family where such expression was taboo. There are only two exercises here for people who are currently dealing with cancer in their lives:

1. Seek a counselor or therapist who is willing to work with you in understanding your feelings of sadness and rage.

2. Find a supportive group (either a cancer support group or a spiritual or community group) where you can express your fears and feelings. Attend it regularly. It is important to be with people who can relate to you. Your family isn't always able to understand completely, although family members can be a valuable support. Take all the help you can get. Be patient with your discovery process. You are traveling new territory in learning about yourself and your feelings. This takes time, but the reward will be worth it.

10
ENERGY: NOT SEEING IS BELIEVING

This is the most mysterious topic of all. For energy can't be seen with the naked eye, although some claim to see human auras and light fields around the human body and other living matter. I have never actually *seen* a human aura. I have, in doing massage, felt an energy field around my clients. Some had energy fields that were so tightly constricted to the body that I almost had to touch the body to feel it. Others seemed to fill the whole room with the energy that emanated from their bodies.

Some scientists say they have captured pictures of this energy through kirlian photography. I tend to be skeptical about the need to take a picture of something I can feel but which is invisible to my naked eye. Nonetheless, much needs to be learned about exactly what this field is. We are just beginning to have a glimmer of understanding.

Without getting esoteric, I admit I made quantum leaps in my own wellness levels when I began to acknowledge and study the mystery of body energy. Many books have been written on the subject. Very little actual scientific evidence exists in the Western world, though the Chinese acupuncturists have been working with it for centuries, as have most of the world's ancient tribal cultures.

We know the body has a healing energy system in and around it; we see the results of what it does, but we have no idea how it works. Medical books show actual photographs of the stages of healing and name the various processes and steps, yet no one really knows how or why healing happens. We just know *that* it happens.

Energy and healing, it seems, are interrelated. Our body cells oscillate at a certain energy level, some higher, some lower. Someday we'll devise an instrument to measure cell oscillation in a way that everyone can understand and accept. (There is a simple instrument that is widely used in Europe and the Orient, although not commonly accredited in Western culture.)

Lower frequency oscillations are the result of energy blockages which come from unexpressed and unrecognized feelings. The result can be, and usually is, illness. Energy blockages also occur when we fail to take action in our lives, or feel trapped in jobs and relationships that are continually painful. Our body energy becomes locked when we feel helpless and hopeless. We are like barometers. When we participate in life fully, our energy goes up; when we allow outside influences to push us around, our energy takes a nosedive. We all have felt highs and lows. These highs and lows, if unattended and ignored, eventually lead to illness.

Does cancer and other disease actually have less chance of occurring when our energy and emotions are flowing freely, when we are not supressing feelings? I believe it does. Dr. Wayne Dyer's *Transformation* audiotapes and Dr. Bernie Siegel's book, *Love, Medicine and Miracles* clearly state that attitudes and beliefs cause and cure disease. It takes time to learn how the principles of healing work, but as you become open to exploring them, you will begin to understand.

Pretend for one day that you actually can use your energy and your mind to create reality around you. See what happens. Affirm in every aspect of your day that you're in charge of how you're feeling. Use your body barometer to tell yourself where the energy is blocked. Think about what could be blocking the energy. Then, visualize yourself taking action in the problem or situation that is obstructing your free energy flow. See how you feel.

If after a day or two of practicing this process you are not convinced of its merit, keep doing it anyway. This is the kind of phenomenon that sneaks up on you one day and turns you into a believer. Don't worry about *making* it happen. When you least expect it you'll be zapped, grabbed by the seat of your hospital gown, and from that moment on, you'll know the truth.

■ ■

ENERGY FIELD EXERCISES

The intent of these exercises is to demonstrate the presence of an energy field around the body that is not visible to the eye. Exactly what this energy is or what it does has not been proven. Record your thoughts on this phenomenon.

1. Find a partner and do the following: Sit in chairs facing each other, knee to knee. Place your left hand facing upward and your right hand facing downward. Ask your partner to do the

same thing, so that your hands are touching; e.g., your left hand, facing upward, lightly touches your partner's right hand, which is facing downward, etc. Sit quietly for a few minutes and see what you experience. Each experience will be different. There is no predicting what will happen. Relax into the time you are spending with your partner and enjoy it! This is not a quiz. There are no right answers.

2. A variation on the above exercise is to stand facing a partner. Each person then takes a step to the left, away from each other. Then place your right hands together, lightly touching. An energy will start to flow between you. Just see where the energy goes, and how the energy seems to move. Again, there is no right or wrong outcome. But you will learn something about yourself in the process. For example, at times your partner will seem to "take control" while other times you will seem to be directing the "flow." Just observe this. Don't try to figure it out.

3. The easiest way to feel another's energy is to sit or stand facing a partner and place one hand about half an inch away from your partner's hand. Slowly move your hands to about 12" away from each other; then gradually move your hands toward each other. Experiment with moving your hand closer and farther from your partner's hand. Record your observations.

4. Without a partner, do the above exercise using your own two hands. You will be amazed at the energy that flows between them!

11
MEDITATION

Meditation comes in all shapes and sizes. To some, meditation means having one's very own mantra or special word that is repeated over and over. Others meditate by seeking total silence within. Massage and athletic sports are forms of meditation that also quiet the mind. The Tibetan monks use ancient song and dance, which include melodic instruments and esoteric vocal toning. Some people call upon guides and dieties. Others use machines and electronic devices to gently slow conscious thought to deep, dream-like states.

The rational mind tends to chatter away constantly, creating feelings of tension and stress in the body. When this chatter is quieted, a miraculous healing occurs. The phenomenon of meditation is considered to be both rejuvenating and regenerating.

To experience this simple and profound state of consciousness (it's a 5000 year old practice), begin by concentrating on your breathing. The Chinese call the breath the "chi." It actually means "life." Inhale to a count of four, hold for two, exhale to four and hold two. Repeat the process for five or ten minutes, building to as much as an hour. The Zen Buddhist monks often meditate for days.

Thousands of books have been written on the subject of

meditation. One particularly delightful paperback is written by a Catholic priest named Anthony deMello, S.J., who blends Christian exercises into Middle Eastern practices. It's called *Sadhana: a Way to God.*.

If you have never meditated before, it may seem strange and even a bit difficult to be still. Your mind will travel and dart to all kinds of thoughts in order to pull you away from the peace you seek. Remember, you are in charge. Stay in the meditation. Gently keep bringing your attention back to the breath. This is the key. It takes practice and good intentions.

The Middle Eastern Indians have an expression that elicits a feeling of oneness with all things when it is spoken: *Namaste* (nah-mas-TAY). As you explore the ancient art of meditation, I wish you peace and love. Namaste!

■■■■■■■■■■■■■■■■■■■■■■■■■■■■■■■

MEDITATION EXERCISES

1. Go to your local modern bookstore and pick up a meditation tape by Louise Hay or Shakti Gawain. Give yourself plenty of time and privacy to listen to the tape, even if you have to lock yourself in a room so you aren't interrupted! It's very important that you make time each day just for YOU! Meditation is a good way to do that.

2. Play a quiet, relaxing musical tape. Seat yourself in a comfortable position, either lying down on the floor (not a bed; you might fall asleep!) or sitting upright in a chair, feet on the floor. Place your hands comfortably in your lap and, with eyes open or closed, begin to pay attention to your breathing. Breathe comfortably and easily for about ten minutes. Begin with short time periods and work your way up to thirty minutes or even an hour. Ideally, choose the same time and place each day to meditate.

3. Record any awarenesses that come to you while meditating, but do it after you have completed your meditation. Sometimes a brilliant idea will come to you while meditating; at other times, silly and trivial thought will run through your mind. Observe them all and just learn to laugh at yourself! We really are quite funny, sometimes, and just as lovable!

4. Play with saying or singing sounds, one syllable, or more, if you wish, until you find one that seems "just right"; e.g., hoo, a-yo, ah-o, iy-ee, etc. You can use this sound current to slide out of the "chatter" mode and into a peaceful one. Using sound actually changes the vibrations of the body.

12
JOURNALING

Journaling can be done at any age; my first experience was at about the age of ten. My Diary (with a capital "D," for it was my friend and confidante) had its own little metal lock and key. I talked to it when no one else would listen. I told it everything. I trusted it to keep my secrets. It contained all my dreams and visions, my anger and fears. I still have it, and as I look at the sometimes tear-stained pages, I wonder what kind of healing took place at that very tender age as I wrote in that book. My Diary is on my list of ten most precious worldly possessions, and I pack it tenderly each time I move to a new home. It goes everywhere with me.

Journaling as I now practice it, is really an extension of my childhood practice. Everything gets journaled, from angry letters that never get mailed to bizarre and revealing dreams. I write to myself, about myself, from myself. My soul is in my journal and all the wisdom of the ages.

Writing actually helps release feelings and thoughts that otherwise would stay locked inside. This releasing process is also very healing, even if your private journal is for your eyes only. Journaling is a way of getting thoughts out of your head and onto the page. It works in much the same way as meditation does.

Journaling will give you a sense of freedom.
There are no rules about how long or how much to journal. Do whatever feels appropriate. Have fun with it. Let your silly self come out, too. Journals don't have to be totally serious. Let your journal be a reflection of all the facets of you. When you publish your journal, as you may someday, send me some of your royalty. I like getting paid for good ideas.

■■■■■■■■■■■■■■■■■■■■■■■■■■■■■■■■■■■■

JOURNALING EXERCISE

Journaling is best done in a quiet place, very early in the day, late at night, or when children are sleeping. This exercise consists of a seven day get-acquainted session of journaling. Each day you will experiment with a different journaling format. At the end of the seventh day, proceed with whatever type of journaling suits you best.

Day 1: Imagine that you have a guide or teacher with whom you wish to communicate. In your journal, write a letter to that guide describing who you are and what is going on with you at this point in your life. Ask your guide some questions or for advice on current dilemmas you may have.

Day 2: Imagine that your guide or teacher is writing you a letter expressing his/her very deep love for you. Allow your guide to comment on the problems or dilemmas which you presented in your journal yesterday.

Day 3: Write a letter to the guardian angel or guide of someone dear to you. It's okay to tell the guide or angel things about that person that may make you angry or sad. Remember, this is your private journal and is not intended to be seen by anyone but you! Say everything that is on your mind, and don't feel guilty about it.

Day 4: Write a letter in your journal addressed directly to a person, living or dead, that you feel angry towards. Don't hold back. Say everything you want to say, including four letter expletives, if necessary. It could be your doctor, a friend, spouse or parent. Let it all out! Don't mail it but notice how you feel when you're finished.

Day 5: Other than expressing feelings, journaling is a powerful tool in recording dreams. Keep your journal by your bed. Record your dreams immediately upon waking, preferably before getting out bed. Better remember to have a pen or pencil next to your journal!

Day 6: Imagine you are writing a letter to yourself when you were about four or five years old. Tell your little self how you feel about him/her and what qualities are the most endearing. Tell your child how much you love him/her and anything else you've always wanted to say.

Day 7: Just for fun, set your alarm for two o'clock in the morning, and journal for half an hour or so about anything that seems fitting.

13
INNER DIALOGUING

Inner dialoguing is simply listening to the inner voice, that voice inside each of us that only has our highest good at heart. It is always loving and supportive, although we don't always like what the inner voice has to say, especially when change is required of us! Inner listening is a process which evolves through many stages until it becomes a finely tuned practice. Once learned, this listening becomes a necessary, even a central part of existence; for closing oneself to our own inner truth, denying that which is best for us, will bring depression, fatigue and, eventually, illness.

All my life I have heard an inner voice guiding me, especially when I got into trouble. It said things like, "Scream bloody murder!" when at the age of ten I got stuck in a tree near my home. Sure enough, an uncle, who heard me from a distance, came and rescued me. Another time my cousin Roger, my dearest friend and confidant at age eleven, got an idea to gather oil from the drums stored for heating in our basement. With it we would light torches from cattails in a nearby swamp. I was both terrified and excited, yet I participated. My inner voice said, "Don't ever do that again. It's dangerous. You might get hurt." My inner self warned me with loving concern. I decided to listen after that.

My inner voice has saved my life many times. It watches out for me when I become distracted or preoccupied with what I think is going to happen in the future. It nudges me back on track when I'm minding somebody else's business. It's the part of me that takes care of me. It has my best interest at heart. Actually, it is the voice of my heart, always knowing what is best for me.

Some give this voice a name. Jose Arguelles, in *Surfers of the Zuvuya*, gives this voice an identity all its own. He calls his guiding voice Uncle Joe. Lee Coit, author of a powerful book called *Listening* describes a step by step plan to access this inner voice and to stay connected with it at all times. An organization called Global Family has as its mission statement a commitment to resonance through the inner listening process. Global Family contends that if each of us is functioning from a place of peace and centeredness, we in turn will reach out to that place of peace and centeredness in others. Global Family is proving the validity of this premise around the globe in places like Russia and Japan with citizen diplomacy programs.

Inner listening is a meditative process. In fact, my first inner guide appeared in a meditation. During a visualization I saw a woman who looked exactly like me, except she was more powerful and more beautiful than I saw myself in real life. I decided to be playful and imaginative, and, in my meditation, I asked her name. She said, "Morgana," and I had a feeling, a sense of truth. Although my rational mind did not believe "Morgana" existed, I continued daily to have conversations with this other side of myself. These dialogues produced beautiful and powerful truths that changed my life. Years later, I learned that the famous psychologist C. G. Jung had an imaginary guide named Philemon, whom Jung credited with most of his creative concepts.

Morgana was my first attempt at getting in touch with that part of myself that knows all things, called the collective unconscious by Carl Jung. Many phases of inner dialoguing with guides may be necessary before the process of going within becomes comfortable. Simply go to a meditative state and ask questions. This requires practice. At first you may get silly or strange answers that don't make sense. Then one day you'll discover that a message was heard but not heeded, like, "Do you have your keys?" and you are now locked out of the house. Some of these "hunches" will make no sense, like Go to this party, or down that street. Yet once you start heeding these hunches, prepare for the exciting and unexpected to happen. Jung calls this synchronicity, the connectedness and meaningfulness of seemingly unrelated events.

The more inner listening you do, the more synchronicity will appear without effort in your life. Taking a playful attitude about each experience will lead to more unexpected delights. Be patient and don't be discouraged if you are not always able to access the inner you. Time is the ultimate teacher and soon you will recognize and trust the inner voice. In fact, you won't make a single decision without being there in the presence of your higher self.

■■■■■■■■■■■■■■■■■■■■■■■■■■■■■■■■■■■■

INNER DIALOGUING EXERCISE

This exercise gives you an opportunity to combine meditation, journaling and inner dialoguing. Inner dialoguing may be done without recording your thoughts or observations; however, to get started, record below any answers that come to you for the following questions. Remember, this takes practice. Also, it's a little tricky to know which of those many voices in our "head" is really our Higher Self—the voice that always knows what's best for us. Don't be discouraged if you're confused at first; with practice you'll begin to recognize your "true voice."

1. Sitting in a quiet place, ask yourself the following question: What do I need to do right now in order to experience joy in my life? Record any answer you may hear inside yourself.

2. Ask: Is there anything you can tell me that will help me understand (describe a situation you want to resolve in your life)? Wait for an answer and record it.

3. Ask: What is the next step I must take in order to achieve (fill in a specific desire) in my life? Record the answer that comes to you.

Once you get the hang of it, you may want to set aside time daily to dialogue without recording the answers. Give your "inner voice" a name if you like, or draw a picture representing that "voice." It could even be represented by an animal or symbol.

14
LIFE'S PURPOSE AND PASSION

"Whatever you can do or dream you can, begin it. Boldness has genius, power and magic in it. Begin it now."
—Goethe

Most of my life has been spent wrestling with the meaning of life. Through three major careers as teacher, corporate executive and massage therapist, I have wondered what was meant by such words as passion and purpose. Joseph Campbell, noted philosopher and humanitarian, says, "Follow your bliss." But, what was my bliss, and how could I follow it if I couldn't find it?

Arnold Patent in his remarkable book, *You Can Have It All*, suggests that "in order to have a life that works perfectly, each of us must be doing what we were created to do—and that is, to express the talent or talents that are given us to express." Patent's wisdom was evasive to me. How could I discover what my talents were until I knew who I was? In my era, little girls grew up to be teachers or nurses. Creativity was discouraged; the creators of the fifties were weirdos and rebels. At least, that's how I saw it.

Getting in touch with my talents and acknowledging them is a fairly recent development for me. As I learn what it is I love to do, an interesting picture emerges. The more I know myself, the more I love myself. The more I love myself, the easier it is to serve others, to give to others. My mission on Earth now becomes: to love myself and to serve others through self love. The details merely become part of the living organism of my existence, growing, changing weekly, daily, hourly. My purpose remains constant: to love.

Have you ever known an auto mechanic or a bus driver who exuded such joy that you couldn't help but be healed in their loving energy? Or a man selling newspapers who, by his mere presence, lets you know he really wants to be there on that particular street corner? Is his task insignificant or unimportant? No matter. He feels wonderful inside, and others feel wonderful in his presence.

If we function from a center of wholeness and self-love, the joy will come through. We will express it from the totality of our being. We will shine!

So, if you find that life's meaning and passion have eluded you, pick a path, any path, and follow it. If you take a few steps and don't like the scenery, pick another path. Keep choosing until you feel "at home," joyful, peaceful. That's it. Persist! You will have arrived at the center of your being, and your passion will emerge like a lover, waiting for you all along, knowing that you'd arrive sooner or later. You will know the truth when you feel the truth. Your heart will tell you. But don't try to hold on to your passion. For it, like you, is ever evolving, ever changing. Allow your passion to flow, to swirl around you, to engulf you. It will give you curiosity and awaken your childlike instincts of wonder and awe. Follow the feeling; flow with it. You will find a synergy that unites body, mind and spirit. And your passion will bring with it a magical gift: Time will become your friend, and it will stand still for you. When all awareness melts into that holy instant of the present moment, you will love self and do whatever expresses that love. That is the passion. That is the gift.

■■■■■■■■■■■■■■■■■■■■■■■■■■■■■■■■■

PURPOSE AND PASSION MEDITATION

This meditation is best done in a comfortable, quiet place. For greater effectiveness, consider recording the meditation in your own voice.

It is a long, long time ago, before you came to the planet Earth. Imagine you are a tiny speck of living matter on a star far, far away. You are aware of a light illuminating you and swirling around inside of you. As the light swirls and moves inside of you, you realize that the light is growing larger and larger, and as the light inside you grows larger and larger, so does your awareness increase. You become aware of the vast distance between you and the other stars and you long to close that distance. You long to become at one with the other stars and planets. As you look out across the vastness of space, your eyes fall upon a beautiful blue pearl, ever so tiny, twirling delicately in space.

And so you make a decision to visit the little Blue Pearl planet because it is so beautiful and you feel a pull of warmth, a longing and desire to be there that becomes so intense that you suddenly become aware that you are moving closer to the Blue Pearl. At first you try to resist, to return to the star of your origin, but the call of the Blue Pearl is so full of love and the promise of adventure that you are unable to resist. You find yourself being irresistibly drawn to the inexpressible joy and warmth of Planet Earth, the Blue Pearl.

*As you approach the planet, you hear the voice of a loving guide, your guide. It asks you to state your reason for choosing to visit Planet Earth. For no one is allowed to enter the protective shield without stating a purpose for the visit. At first you become uncomfortable about being asked such a question, but you soon realize that **only you** can decide on a purpose; so you ask "What is my purpose?" And you wait. [Pause.] You also realize that you can make the visit as much fun and as exciting as you want it to be. So you smile and a picture begins to form, a picture with you in it. Through a mist you see yourself in your present state. You are doing joyful and interesting activities, full of fun and adventure. Take a moment to see yourself in this picture. [Pause.] You are not alone. Other loving people are with you and you realize that you are together as a team in many loving activities. A feeling of great peace fills you as you become aware of how very much you are loved by those around you. You are filled with gratitude for all your teammates and you feel the happiness inside you. [Pause.]*

Soon you awaken in a small, grassy field on a hillside. You sit up, look around you, take a deep breath of the cool, clear air and rise to your feet, which are very strong and able to support your healthy body. You begin your adventure with a sense of wonder and curiosity, keenly aware of your direction, yet open to all the surprises and changes along the way.

15
THE DOCTOR OF THE FUTURE

> *"The doctor of the future will give no medicine but will interest his patients in the care of the human frame, in diet, and in the cause and prevention of disease."*
>
> —*Thomas A. Edison*

The great American inventor, Thomas Edison, had a vision for wellness. Edison saw doctors *assisting* their patients in devising their own wellness formulas. It is not an impossible dream. In fact, patient responsibility is a necessary step for healing the current state of affairs in the medical community; namely, the stressed out doctors and nurses who are faltering under the awesome responsibility they have assumed for the maintenance of human life. We expect the medical community to save us from our own indulgences, which include countless forms of addictions and self-abuse. Many of us look to doctors to be "fixed" or "cured." And doctors have willingly taken on the task of rescuer and even savior. But this system isn't working. Nurses are leaving their profession in droves, burned out and disillusioned. Doctors awaken in the middle of the night with a burning urge to get back to the hospital, overwhelmed with feelings of incompletion and helplessness.

Recently I met and talked with doctors at a medical convention. Several doctors expressed an interest in and even related positive personal experiences with alternative health practices such as massage and acupuncture. There was a general willingness of doctors to know more about practices such as visualization. Doctors appeared willing to experience massage themselves and even prescribed it for their patients. Many expressed an interest in exploring circumstances and situations where massage could be used as an adjunct to the patient's medical treatment. Some told me they had massage therapists on duty in their clinics. I felt hopeful. The construction of the bridge between the medical profession and the alternative health care professions is very much underway and becoming more and more evident. There's much to be done in educating the public and increasing communication between doctors and alternative health care professionals, but progress is being made.

Sadly enough, these men and women are tired and in poor health themselves. Many are overweight. Could it be that they are wounded healers, themselves needing help and support? Are they nurturing themselves or are they trying to accomplish superhuman tasks in caring for others because we have come to expect it of them? These questions point up a challenge for each of us: to act altruistically in caring for our health and our life and to use the medical profession as teachers and guides only.

Edison's expansive vision means this: That each and every one of us has the personal responsibility to become our own doctor, to sharpen our intuitive senses, our knowledge of self, to the extent that we know our bodies, quite literally, inside and out. We need to discover what our bodies need to thrive, not just survive. We have an injunction to respect our own physicalness not only for its own sake, but because our bodies contain mental and spiritual aliveness as well.

Those of us who have allowed the body to become sick to a point where medical help is required must acknowledge that we have gone beyond the point of self help. In that case, we must go quickly to our doctor of choice and cooperate fully with his or her suggestions for recovery. Manifesting actual symptoms of disease is evidence enough that this is not the time to experiment with non-medical alternatives. I do, however, recommend using alternative medicine in conjunction with your doctor's treatment. Combining medical procedures with alternative healing practices is exponentially a winning combination.

The bottom line is, you alone and not your doctor's prognosis, determines whether you live or die, and how and when. It's a lot of responsibility, but it's one that the doctors never wanted in the first place.

Eleven years ago I received the pathology report as I sat in a hospital bed following my lung surgery, removal of a tumor in the lower lobe of my right lung. "Inconclusive," the report stated. My doctor explained that the cell study of the tumor suggested it could be either Hodgkins, a relatively slow-growing cancer, or oat cell carcinoma, in which case I'd be dead in six months. The vote by four pathologists was tied, 2 to 2. *I* cast the deciding vote. With my ever-present sense of humor, I figured that if I was going to be given a choice, I'd choose the kinder of the two options. I also purposely chose to decide that the tumor had been removed completely and that I'd never have cancer again.

On a very deep level I chose to live, but I didn't have a clue what living meant or how I would take my first baby steps back to health. I had my own unique set of stumbling blocks and, in retrospect, it's just as well I didn't have a crystal ball back in 1978. For the road to peace and empowerment was paved with great resistance on my part. Taking responsibility for my own wellness was a commitment and, once begun, there was no turning back.

If you make a commitment to life—YOURS—you still may not be clear about your path, or how you're going to get from a hospital bed to a ski slope. But if you haven't guessed by now: the Doctor of the Future is, in the truest sense, none other than YOU!

16
COMMITMENT

It takes dogged determination and stamina to nurture a weak and fragile body back to robustness and vigor. When I completed radiation therapy 11 years ago, the radiologist promised me longevity. The thought both thrilled and jarred me. I had been preparing to die, and now I was being told I could expect to live twice as long as I already had! At that point, dying almost seemed like an easier option. For, in truth, I didn't know *how* to live, not in a joyful, productive way. Not with awareness and a sense of purpose.

Would I do things differently? Could I change belief systems and behavior patterns I had identified with since birth? What did taking charge of my life really entail? Would I take responsibility for this "holy temple," my body, which until recently seemed to be dying? Could I shift my intentions and dedicate myself to health and life? And where would I begin?

The only clue I had was the hope of the radiologist's words. Many times since then, when I doubted I would stay healthy, when fear of recurrence gripped me, I would remember the doctor's prophesy. And that hope would sustain me.

I went on living. Through psychotherapy, reading positive books, skiing, running, swimming, teaching fitness classes and support groups, my fantasies began to materialize. Life became little victory after little victory, though not always easy. Daily, hourly, second by second, commitment to optimal health was required. Sometimes my body would warn me with mysterious aches and pains. Body signs have a way of getting me back on track, a reminder to take care of myself. My body barometer of pain was always a clue that something needed attention, that I was getting out of touch with myself. The checklist in my head itemized the possible origin of my physical discomfort: Was it my job, a relationship, emotional denial, my children or my parents that was bugging me?

Believe it or not, a pain in the elbow the day your boss gives you a huge assignment with an unreasonable deadline could mean you're angry. Talking to your boss can make the pain disappear as quickly as it occurred. Try taking action in your life whenever you have some physical pain. Make it a game. When body discomfort appears, figure out who or what needs to be dealt with. Invariably the discomfort will disappear when you *do something* concrete instead of just mulling.

My younger daughter recently told me she used this technique with a canker sore that appeared in her mouth. She realized she needed to tell her father that the radio he bought her for Christmas wasn't working properly. As soon as she moved through the discomfort of telling her dad, the canker sore disappeared.

The connection between disease and feelings (and, more importantly, the action we take in our lives once we acknowledge our feelings) is becoming widely recognized. Experimenting with body discomforts in this way will amaze and amuse you.

What's more, it costs less than a pharmaceutical prescription and works faster! Begin practicing this technique on little ailments rather than major afflictions. Start small, when you are reasonably healthy. If you aren't in good health, remember to take help from all sources. Don't play games with yourself once serious disease has manifested in your body. That's the time you may need big guns: like surgery, radiation, chemotherapy, experimental drugs. Your belief systems got you sick in the first place. Changing them is like turning a battleship around in the ocean. It takes time and commitment.

It may be difficult to confront loved ones with your needs and wishes, but it is a very necessary part of your wellness formula. As you experiment with asking for what you want, you may discover that often the pain you feel is in your expectations of others. World leader and philosopher Mahatma Ghandi, when asked for a formula for living simply said, "Renounce, and do." It is essential to release expectations and attachments regarding others and to act responsibly according to your own needs for fulfillment.

Living another thirty-five years is a very appealing thought. Somewhere along the way, I signed up to live. It seems the choice to live or die is something we do with every breath we take. Each second becomes a choice, a decision.

Olympic athletes serve as a model for grit and dedication to excellence. These youths demonstrate passion with every move; goals and visions shine in their eyes. They are aglow with intention; nothing distracts them. Preventing and recovering from illness requires the same approach. We must set goals and focus on the vision of radiant health and joy.

Stepping off the path with a chocolate bar or a Big Mac may happen occasionally. Sometimes a nagging headache reminds me of an unresolved gripe I have with a dear friend. That is when the little voice gets bigger and stronger and yanks me back on the path. Again I feel my body with its health and wholeness. Again I dedicate and rededicate myself to the sacred task of enjoying my physicalness.

The ancient Sufis of the Middle East have an expression that serves as a motto: *Ya Hayy, Ya Haqq*, (Ya HIGH, Ya HUCK). O Life, O Truth. As you dedicate yourself to living, in truth, to your highest potential, I salute you. Ya Hayy, Ya Haqq!

SELECTED BIBLIOGRAPHY

Arguelles, Jose, *Surfers of the Zuvuya*, Bear & Co., 1989.

Campbell, T. C., quoted in Lang, S., "Diet and Disease," *Food Monitor*, May/June, 1983, p. 24, as quoted by Robbins, John, *Diet for a New America*.

Coit, Lee, *Listening*, Las Brisas Retreat Center, 1985.

deMello, Anthony, S.J., *Sadhana: A Way to God*, The Institute of Jesuit Sources, 1978.

Diamond, Harvey and Marilyn, *Fit for Life*, Warner Books, Inc., 1985.

Dyer, Wayne, *Transformation: You'll See It When You Believe It*, audiotape produced by Nightingale-Conant, 1987.

Global Family, 112 Jordan Avenue, San Anselmo, CA 94960. Telephone 415-453-7600.

Haas, Robert, *Eat to Win*, Signet, 1983.

Nicholson, Shirley, ed., *Shamanism: An Expanded View of Reality*, Theosophical Publishing House, 1987.

Patent, Arnold, *You Can Have It All*, Celebration Publishing, 1984.

Robbins, John, *Diet for a New America*, Stillpoint Publishing, 1987.

Siegel, Bernie S., *Love, Medicine & Miracles*, Harper & Row, 1986.

Simonton, O. Carl and Stephanie, *Getting Well Again*, J.P. Tarcher, Inc., 1978.

Winick, M., quoted in Goodman, D., "Breaking the Protein Myth," *Whole Life Times*, July/August, 1984, p.26, as quoted by Robbins, John, *Diet for a New America*.

ABOUT THE AUTHOR

Jan King Garverick is a wellness lecturer and workshop leader. She has taught high school and has also spent ten years as a business professional at Zenith Electronics, where she specialized in the international marketplace.

Pottery is one of her latest fascinations, along with daily yoga practice.

Ms. Garverick resides in Evanston, Illinois, and has two adult daughters, Nicole and Trina Goetz.

SELF-HEALING DYNAMICS

by Jan King Garverick

Give a gift of health to your friends!

ORDER FORM

Morgana Publications
P. O. Box 5403
Evanston, IL 60204 - 5403

Please send me:

_____ copies of **Self-Healing Dynamics**
$7.95 plus $1.00 postage and handling.
(Illinois residents add sales tax of $.49 per book)
Quantity discounts for 10 or more at $5.00 each
plus tax, postage and handling.

Enclosed is $_____.
(Check or money order; no cash or C.O.D. please.)

Name: _____

Address: _____

City: _____ State: _____ Zip: _____

Telephone: _____